HOW TO HANG UP
YOUR HANG-UPS:
The Power of God's Grace

By

Dr. Rufus E. Medlin

ACKNOWLEDGEMENTS

I thank God the Father, God the son and God the Holy Spirit for giving me the grace, wisdom and a successful career in counseling and psychiatry practice that has resulted in the publication of this book.

I also want to thank my wife, Dell for the mighty woman of God and a devoted wife that she is to me. You have been one of my greatest blessings. Thank you Dell.

I thank my daughter and her family for their love and support. You are my joy.

HOW TO HANG UP YOUR HANG-UPS:
The Power of God's Grace

All scriptures are quoted from the King James and
Amplified Versions of the Bible.

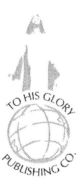

Published by: To His Glory Publishing Company, Inc.
463 Dogwood Drive
Lilburn, GA 30047
(770) 458-7947
www.tohisglorypublishing.com

Book is available at:
Amazon.com, BarnesandNoble.com, Borders.com,
Booksamillion.com etc.
www.tohisglorypublishing.com
(770) 458-7947

Cover designed by: To His Glory Publishing Co.

International Standard Book Number: **0-9749802-9-3**

DEDICATION

I dedicate this book to God the Father, God the Son and God the Holy Ghost. Lord God, You gave me the words to write in this book and I give you all the glory.

I also dedicate this book to my wife Dell and my daughter Diane Tietz and her family.

I wish to dedicate this book also to Clarietha Allen and Jennye Guy.

FOREWORD

Dr. Medlin has provided a tremendous work of wisdom for those who want to get rid of their hang-ups and help others do the same. Dr. Medlin's educational background and years of work as a psychiatrist plus his Biblical knowledge of God's divine principles make this a vital contribution to all who desire deliverance and transformation. God bless you, Rufus, for making these workable truths known to us.

-Dr. Bill Hamon
Chairman, Founder and Bishop of Christian
International Ministries Network

TABLE OF CONTENTS

PREFACE

As we mature, we all realize, sooner or later, that we have **"hang-ups,"** those little idiosyncrasies that make us distinct; those "difficult" things that we have to cope with; those things that are hard for us to understand and overcome. They hinder, they bind and they "hang us up" so that we cannot reach our potential as individuals. If we could free ourselves from these hang-ups, the world would be a much better place in which to live, and we would enjoy living much more than we do.

These hang-ups come from many different sources. We are truly the product of all our experiences as well as our genetic inheritance. This combination—character, behavior, dreams, ambitions and philosophy—makes us what we are: As we go through life, the hard knocks produce hurts and bruises; the positive, good experiences produce growth and love. All of this comes from human relationships.

In the process of relating to each other we "rub off" the rough spots or blemishes and heal the bruises, hurts and hard knocks. If we live according to the principles laid down in God's Word, we come out of all these experiences better people because we have benefited from God's grace—a grace that not only flows from God to us, but from God's children to us as well.

As we are shaped, bent, fitted and fashioned by the forces that God brings to lean on us, we can truly become God-like individuals. If you study the life of Christ, you are quickly struck by the fact that though he was God, he was indeed man. Just like you and I, He experienced all the emotions, all the temptations, all the negatives and all the positives during his life here on earth. He was pretty much like you and me. He, too, had to grow and mature to a point before his ministry started. He continued to grow and mature even after the beginning of his ministry. His life made a difference in his world.

So, too, you and I can live lives that make a difference. Long after we are gone, our lives can testify that the world was made a better place because we lived.

- Dr. Rufus E. Medlin

HANG-UP NUMBER ONE:
Who Has the Answer?

Down through the centuries, man has sought to explain his woes, hang-ups and emotional problems in various ways. There seems to be a prevalent notion that we know so much more than our forefathers that somehow their knowledge, abilities, and explanations of events fall far short of our insights and knowledge. I'm sure that in many, many instances this is true; in others, I'm not so sure.

A great deal of psychological and psychiatric thought has contributed to our current beliefs, ideas and practice. Much of this body of knowledge consists of man's efforts to look within himself and find answers to his needs and to what makes him tick. Where else would you look? However, there is more than intellect involved in trying to find these answers. It is like trying to pull yourself up by your own bootstraps: You cannot do it. All of man's emotional and psychological cures cannot be found within himself.

Freud usually gets much attention, although there were many men before him who influenced psychiatric thought. Freud's method of releasing repressed ideas is expressed as catharsis, or free association. He is also known for his work on dream analysis, the hypothesis of the unconscious, and studies of the stages of psychosexual development. These theories, along with his studies of the psychopathology of every day life and the analysis of transference reactions, form the historical basis for much of modern psychotherapy.

There were others besides Freud who made significant contributions to psychiatric thought. Here are a few of them.

Jung wrote of word associations, personality types and psychological aspects of man's religious and cultural

15

strivings (the collective unconscious).

There was Adler, who broke away from Freud to form his own school which promulgated theories of individual psychology, including a theory of aggression producing neurotic symptoms and resulting from organ inferiority. His simple formulations such as "inferiority complex" had great popular appeal.

Adolph Meyer, the dean of American psychiatry, presented the broad concepts of psychobiology. He focused the psychiatrist's attention upon the total context of the social, emotional and physical basis of personality and introduced the life chart and distributive analysis.

Then there was Paul Schilder and his body image concepts. Harry Stack Sullivan thought personality developed in response to family patterns of social interaction. He also believed that anxiety is basically a feature of a relationship rather than that of an individual. He stressed the therapist's role as a participant observer in the patient's system of disturbed relationships.

With the advent of pharmacology and psychoactive drugs, it was shown that many aspects of behavior, disturbed thought and emotions, had a biological basis. With the production and use of CAT and PET scanners and various investigative, diagnostic and physiologic techniques, it becomes more apparent that disordered function is associated with disordered behavior.

Where does God fit into all of this? It would appear that the many methods, treatments and remedies work only some of the time at best, and that cures are few and far between. This lets us know that many of our methods are hit and miss efforts. We cannot pull ourselves up by our own bootstraps. <u>There has to be another answer</u>.

That is where God comes in. He is the answer. God made man. Since He made man, He understands him and knows how to heal him.

If we look into the Word of God, we can find answers to our problems and needs in our lives, our families, and our businesses. The Bible says, "What is man that thou art mindful of him?" The answer comes that man was created as a God-class of being by God and for God's pleasure. Through the Lord Jesus Christ, you and I can know God intimately.

In God's Word we find principles for us to live by. If we use them we can be very successful, happy, and content. The 1st Psalm describes what happens to a man who honors God and walks in His ways: "He shall be like a tree planted by the rivers of water, that brings forth his fruit in his season, his leaf also shall not wither, and whatsoever he doeth shall prosper."

This is a far cry from what we see today in people's lives. The answer to man's problems in this greatly enlightened world of ours is not within ourselves. It is not a method. It is not a theory. It is not a practice—but a person, the Lord Jesus Christ. In Him dwells all the fullness of God. We can have a relationship with Him simply by asking Him to come into our lives and become Lord.

What does the Bible say about this relationship? We find the answers in the following scriptures.

Romans 5:8
"But God commanded His love toward us, in that, while we were yet sinners, Christ died for us."

John 3:16
"For God so loved the world, that He gave His only begotten Son, that whosoever believeth in Him should not perish, but have everlasting life."

John 14:27

"Peace I leave with you, my peace I give unto you: not as the world giveth, give I unto you. Let not your heart be troubled, neither let it be afraid."

II Corinthians 5:17

"Therefore if any man be in Christ, he is a new creature: old things are passed away; behold, all things are become new."

II Corinthians 5:21

"For he hath made him to be sin for us, who knew no sin; that we might be made the righteousness of God in him."

I Corinthians 1:9

"God is faithful, by whom ye were called unto the fellowship of his son Jesus Christ Our Lord."

I Peter 2:21

"For even hereunto were ye called: because Christ also suffered for us, leaving us an example, that ye should follow his steps."

II Thessalonians 3:3

"But the Lord is faithful, who shall stablish you, and keep you from evil."

Philippians 4:19

"But my God shall supply all your need according to his riches in glory by Christ Jesus."

Psalm 37:4
"Delight thyself also in the Lord; and he shall give thee the desires of thine heart."

II Timothy 3:16-17
"All scripture is given by inspiration of God, and is profitable for doctrine, for reproof, for correction, for instruction in righteousness: That the man of God may be perfect, throughly furnished unto all good works."

These are but a few of the scriptures that point us to God as the answer for most of our problems. As we commit ourselves to God and His service, it becomes evident to us rather quickly what course our lives should take. Whatever we are, whatever our occupation, serving God aligns us with forces that are unstoppable. Studying God's Word provides us with life principles to live by. Communication with God reveals how we can help others to be happy and become more successful. This adds up to a new way of life that is very satisfying, and full of excitement and adventure. Can you ask for more than that? Try it; you will like it.

Basically, this is the way to hang up your Hang-ups but let us also examine our other hang-ups more closely.

HANG-UP NUMBER TWO:
Loneliness

All of us have been lonely at times. In fact, loneliness is often called "The Most Common Malady Known to Man."

WHAT IS LONELINESS?

Loneliness is a painful awareness that we lack meaningful contact with others. It involves a feeling of inner emptiness, and may be accompanied by sadness, discouragement, a sense of isolation, unworthiness, anxiety, and an intense desire to be wanted or needed. Lonely, depressed people feel like they are of little worth.

KINDS OF LONELINESS

1. Emotional – the lack or loss of intimate relationships with another person or persons. These people need to renew in-depth relationships with others.
2. Social – a feeling of aimlessness, anxiety and emptiness. This individual feels that he or she is "out of it." These people need support from accepting friends, either one-on-one or in groups.
3. Spiritual – the sense of isolation experienced by a person who is separated from God and feels that he/she has no meaning or purpose in life.

SOLITUDE AND LONELINESS

What is the difference between solitude and loneliness? Solitude can be refreshing, rejuvenating and enjoyable. Everyone needs times when they can be alone to commune with just themselves. Times of solitude tend to renew and give us a different look on life. On the other hand, loneliness is painful, draining and unpleasant.

CAUSES OF LONELINESS

There are a variety of causes of loneliness. Let's take a look at some of them:

1. Social

Rapid social changes, such as we see in our world today, tend to isolate people from each other.

2. Technology

As this gets greater, people tend to feel smaller, less important or less needed. Efficiency and convenience become more important and there is less time for developing meaningful relationships with others.

3. Mobility

We are living in a world that is very mobile. The average family moves five times every two years.

4. Urbanization

As people have moved closer together, there has come a distrust of strangers; thus suspicion, withdrawal and loneliness.

5. Television

This stops communication as well as relationships and causes loneliness.

6. Arrested or Incomplete Development

There are three basic developmental needs that must be met if loneliness is to be avoided:

    a. Attachment – We need to feel a closeness, a bond, to others.

    b. Acceptance – Children need to be accepted by their parents. Adults need to be accepted by their peers. Low self-esteem often prevents us from relating to others or being accepted by others.

    c. Social Skills – All of us need to acquire social skills to build solid, smooth interpersonal relationships.

7. Psychological Causes

These include low self-esteem, hostility, fear, self defeating attitudes, and the inability to communicate.

8. Situational Causes

These include circumstances experienced by those who are single, widowed, living alone, grieving, elderly, etc. People in leadership positions sometimes are lonely. Because they feel they are different, persons who are physically disabled or diseased may be lonely.

9. Spiritual Causes

These are rather common. We may feel lonely if we rebel spiritually and reject God. Many seek meaning in drugs, sex, work, sports and many other things.

When this happens and we neglect our
relationship with God, we may become
lonely.

WHAT CAN BE DONE ABOUT LONELINESS?

Many suggestions are offered for the cure
of loneliness, from changing jobs to developing new
hobbies. These may work to some degree. Loneliness   is
a spiritual problem, however, and we need to deal with
it on a much deeper level. Here is a list of things to do in
order to cope with loneliness:

1. Admit that we have it.
2. Decide to do something about it.
3. Consider the cause or causes.
4. Accept what cannot be changed.
5. Change what can be changed, such as:
a. Develop self-esteem
b. Take some risks – (for example, reach out to others
or risk "getting involved")
6. Develop social skills.
You can do this by seeking help from a counselor or
by reading books.
7. Get your spiritual needs met.
We need human companionship; but more than that,
we need a relationship with God. If we know Him,
we have a way of dealing with loneliness through the
Word of God, the person of Jesus Christ and the Holy
Spirit.

What does the Bible say that will help us stop
loneliness? Here are some appropriate scripture references.
Psalm 139:7
"Whither shall I go from thy Spirit? or whither shall I flee
from thy presence?"

Hebrews 13:5
"For God Himself has said, I will not in any way fail you nor give you up nor leave you without support. I will not, I will not, I will not in any degree leave you helpless nor forsake, nor let you down (relax my hold on you) assuredly not!"

John 14:23
"If a man love me, he will keep my words; and my father will love him, and we will come unto him and make our abode with him."

Isaiah 41:10
"Fear thou not; for I am with thee: be not dismayed; for I am thy God: I will strengthen thee; yea, I will help thee; yea, I will uphold thee with the right hand of my righteousness."

Joshua 1:9
"Have not I commanded thee? Be strong and of a good courage; be not afraid neither be thou dismayed: for the Lord thy God is with thee whithersoever thou goest."

Let the Lord fill you with His Holy Spirit. The Holy Spirit is a teacher, an advocate, a helper, one who is called alongside us to help us. He will live inside you and be a source of strength in every circumstance. As **John 14:26** says, "He shall teach you all things, and bring all things to your remembrance."

A vibrant relationship with the Lord Jesus Christ will cure your loneliness and set you free, allowing you to hang up this Hang-up and attain a level of successful living that you could never reach otherwise.

SOME PERSONAL OBSERVATIONS

I would like to share a couple of personal experiences from the days when I maintained a psychiatric practice. These stories show how, if you will trust God and look to Him, then He will help you, whatever your circumstance might be. He will answer prayer, meet your needs, and help you change your life. It will take effort on your part, as well as from family members and others who are willing to help you make the change. But change can be achieved.

I treated a man for alcoholism when he was a patient at the VA Hospital in Columbia, South Carolina. While undergoing treatment, the Lord came into his heart and my patient was born again. He completed treatment and I didn't see him again until 12 years later. He told me that he became a Christian while at the hospital and had not taken a drop of alcohol since then.

Another one of my patients at the hospital had what is called a manic depressive psychosis. With care and treatment by my treatment team and me, the patient was able to settle down. He, too, gave his heart to the Lord and began to serve God while he was under my care. After he was released, I saw him on several occasions when he came back for checkups. He had to remain on medication but he got along fine with God's help.

These patients, and others like them whose changes I have witnessed, show the power of Christ to move in situations when people submit themselves to Him.

Dr. Rufus E. Medlin

HANG-UP NUMBER THREE
Depression

For more than 2,500 years depression has been recognized as a common problem. Many years ago, it was called melancholia. Depression is mentioned in connection with Saul, Israel's first king. Saul had a rather wide, prolonged mood swings. Today we would call him a manic-depressive with a cyclic pattern. From what is related to us about him in scripture, it appears that he would have episodes of elation as well as episodes of depression. David would play the harp for Saul and the music would quiet his spirit.

Depression has become so commonly recognized and has received so much attention that many people are calling this the "age of depression" or the "era of melancholy"—in contrast to the "age of anxiety" that followed WWII.

Depression varies from the temporary symptoms of sadness and general debility associated with the loss of a loved one to the much deeper suicidal depression of a psychotic. Signs of depression include sadness, apathy, inability to make decisions, low self-esteem, feelings of worthlessness and helplessness along with feelings of guilt and shame. There is also a loss of interest in work or sex, loss of appetite, poor bowel function, difficulty in concentrating and lack of spontaneity. Depression can occur at any age, even in infants.

TYPES OF DEPRESSION

There are different types of depression:

Reactive -- usually associated with a great loss or some great life trauma; **Endogenous** -- usually

27

seen in middle-aged and older individuals and characterized by its depth and difficulty to treat;

Psychotic -- usually involves intense despair, self- destructive thoughts and/or attempts, hallucinations and loss of contact with reality;

Neurotic -- usually associated with much anxiety, it is much easier to treat.

These brief descriptions show that depression is complex, is often difficult to treat, and can be very perplexing at times.

THE CAUSES OF DEPRESSION

Depression has many causes, some of which appear to be related to disordered physiology, while others seem to be related entirely to events that have happened in one's life. Understanding the causes of depression can help us deal with it.

Physical Causes
1. Loss of sleep
2. Improper diet
3. Side effects of drugs
4. Low blood sugar or Hypoglycemia
5. Brain tumors
6. Glandular disorders such as those related to the hypothalamus and its functioning

Early Experiences
   Some researchers say that childhood experiences can cause depression in later life.
Learned Helplessness
   Some researchers say that repeated encountering of

situations that you have no control over can cause you to adopt an attitude of helplessness. We become depressed when we learn that all our efforts are futile.

Loss

Loss of a loved one or some loved object— home, business, fortune, family, friends, etc.—can cause depression.

Negative Thinking

We are programmed by society toward negative thinking, to see the dark side and overlook the brighter side. This practice can lead to depression and probably contributes to the widespread prevalence of depression. According to psychiatrist Aaron Beck, people show negative thinking predominantly in three areas:

1. They view the world and their life experiences negatively.
2. Life is seen as a series of defeats in a world that is fast going down the tube.
3. Most depressed people feel they are inadequate, unworthy and incapable of performing in an adequate manner. They have a low self-image or self-esteem. Just as they view the past and the present in a negative way, they see the future in the same light: i.e., it is hopeless, frustrating, and filled with difficulties that are insolvable.

Stress

Life's stresses can stimulate depression. Job stress can cause depression.

Anger

The oldest known cause of depression is anger that is

turned on the self. Many homes, schools, and workplaces will not tolerate the expression of anger. Anger bottled up over a period of years can result in depression.

Hurt, anger, and revenge expressed one of three ways:
1. Destructive actions
2. Psychosomatic symptoms
3. Depression

Hurt can arise from a direct offense by someone or through disappointment. Most people react to these hurts with anger or resentment. To hide the hurt, they express more anger. Oftentimes, a desire for revenge will help cover up anger, leading to destructive or violent acts.

Covering up anger can lead to "shoving it down" our gastrointestinal tract, resulting in psychosomatic complaints because we can't "stomach" all that hurt. Or we become depressed, turning our anger on ourselves. All of this hiding from anger takes tremendous amounts of energy and wears down our body. We may consciously, or even unconsciously, condemn ourselves for our negative feelings and anger. This makes us more depressed.

Guilt

Another great producer of depression is guilt. It is easy to see how this works: Self-condemnation produces feelings of worthlessness and hopelessness which, in turn, breed depression.

Satanic Influence

The devil does attack God's children. One of his cruel, oppressive devices is despondence and depression. We must recognize that often depression is an attack of Satan. Through prayer and intercession, the sufferer can be delivered by God. As believers, we have authority bestowed on us by Jesus, our Lord, to cast Satan out in these instances.

THE EFFECTS OF DEPRESSION

Some of the effects of depression are unhappiness, inefficiency, hidden or masked reactions, withdrawal, and suicide.

All depressives are unhappy. Most feel blue, unwanted, unloved, hopeless and very self-critical. These people usually have little enthusiasm. They are indecisive, and have very little energy for doing even simple tasks. They are usually underachievers and become increasingly dependent on other people.

In some, their denial works so well that they succeed in hiding their depression from themselves. As a result, they develop all kinds of psychosomatic symptoms and syndromes. They may mask their depression through impulsive acts, temper outbursts, acts of aggression or destructiveness, being accident prone, gambling, drinking, exhibiting compulsive work habits and having sexual problems. Suicide is the ultimate way to escape the ravages of depression. Suicide and suicide attempts are seen more often in teenagers, people living alone, and unmarried or divorced persons.

All of the above show the pervasiveness and destructive effects of depression on peoples' lives. These effects will be seen often by anyone who treats or counsels the depressed.

DEALING WITH DEPRESSION

There are many ways that we deal with depression. Based on what we know about this disorder's characteristics, we can spot depression if we suspect it in those who come to us for help. This requires that we be good listeners and that we ask the right questions to get confirming information.

Depressives need tender love and care and it requires much patience and understanding to help them. The Holy Spirit can help us recognize depression's symptoms, ask the right questions and offer understanding and support while encouraging the depressive to be responsible and willing to deal with the problem he or she faces.

One way to deal with depression is to refer the sufferer to a psychiatric clinic where medical treatment of the depression can be instituted; many depressions will require this action.

Another way to deal with depression, if it is determined that suicide is not a risk, is to evaluate the depressed person and ascertain a cause. Deal with the cause that you find by using scripture and the insights afforded by the Holy Spirit. Sin, revenge, unforgiveness, anger and hurts, must all be dealt with in an appropriate manner in order to rid someone of his feelings of depression.

You <u>can</u> control your mind—it belongs to you. **Philippians 4:8** is a good scripture reference to use: "Finally, brethren, whatsoever things are true, whatsoever things are honest, whatsoever things are just, whatsoever things are pure, whatsoever things are lovely, whatsoever things are of good report; if there be any virtue, and if there be any praise, think on these things." This is also a good reference scripture for the depressed person.

Many times, people who are depressed must be protected from themselves. We should never fail to do this. Here are some keys that indicate when protection should be given:

    1. Excessive concern about physical illness

    2. Any evidence to suggest a plan for suicide or talk of suicide

3. Preoccupation with insomnia
4. Expressions of feelings of hopelessness
5. Feelings of worthlessness and extreme guilt
6. A sudden change in mood from depression to happiness
7. Any inclination of "giving up" or resigning oneself to failure

One should not hesitate to talk about these characteristics and to question a person about their feelings on suicide. Open discussion could conceivably reduce the likelihood of suicide. Sometimes you can make a pact or agreement that the person will not do it until he contacts you and has an opportunity to discuss his plan with you.

If, during your experience as a counselor, you are involved in a potential suicide situation, be supportive and take decisive action by getting the individual to a psychiatrist or a psychiatric facility.

THE BIBLE AND DEPRESSION

There are many references to depression and grieving in the Word of God. The term depression is not used since this is a clinical term, but depression is certainly implied. **Three Psalms—69, 88, and 102**—are songs of despair, but they are set in a context of hope.

Jeremiah, the weeping prophet, wrote the book of Lamentations. Elijah, the mighty prophet of Israel, saw God work in a miraculous way on Mt. Carmel, but then fled from Jezebel's threats into the wilderness where he became despondent. Elijah felt the depths of despair and wanted to die. God intervened in a miraculous way to spare Elijah's life.

Jesus in Gethsemane is another example. He was burdened with such grief and sadness that brought so much stress that he sweat drops of blood.

In spite of all the despair and sadness in these

examples, their basic theme is hope that is carried by a strong faith in God and His faithfulness to His children.

Reference scriptures on depression and hope include the following:

Psalm 34:17

"The righteous cry, and the Lord heareth, and delivereth them out of all their troubles."

Isaiah 43:2

"When thou passest through the waters, I will be with thee; and through the rivers, they shall not overflow thee: When thou walkest through the fire, thou shalt not be burned; neither shall the flame kindle upon thee."

Romans 8:38-39

"For I am persuaded, that neither death, nor life, nor angels, nor principalities, nor powers, nor things present, nor things to come, nor height, nor depth, nor any other creature, shall be able to separate us from the love of God, which is in Christ Jesus our Lord."

Psalm 147:3

"He healeth the broken in heart, and bindeth up their wounds."

Isaiah 51:11

"Therefore the redeemed of the Lord shall return, and come with singing unto Zion; and everlasting joy shall be upon their head: they shall obtain gladness and joy; and sorrow and mourning shall flee away."

Mark 16:16-18

"He that believeth and is baptized shall be saved; but he that believeth not shall be damned. And these signs shall follow them that believe; In my name shall they cast out devils; they shall speak with new tongues; They shall take up serpents; and if they drink any deadly thing, it shall not hurt them; they shall lay hands on the sick, and they shall recover."

Luke 10:17-19

"And the seventy returned again with joy, saying, Lord, even the devils are subject unto us through thy name. And he said unto them, I beheld Satan as lightning fall from heaven. Behold, I give unto you power to tread on serpents and scorpions, and over all the power of the enemy: and nothing shall by any means hurt you."

Matthew 12:28-29

"But if I cast out devils by the Spirit of God, then the kingdom of God is come unto you. Or else how can one enter into a strong man's house, and spoil his goods, except he first bind the strong man? and then he will spoil his house."

II Corinthians 10:3-5

"For though we walk in the flesh, we do not war after the flesh: (For the weapons of our warfare are not carnal, but mighty through God to the pulling down of strongholds;) Casting down imaginations, and every high thing that exalteth itself against the knowledge of God, and bringing into captivity every thought to the obedience of Christ."

Ephesians 6:10-18

"Finally, my brethren, be strong in the Lord, and in the power of his might. Put on the whole armour of God, that ye may be able to stand against the wiles of the devil. For we wrestle not against flesh and blood, but against principalities, against powers, against the rulers of the darkness of this world, against spiritual wickedness in high places. Wherefore take unto you the whole armour of God, that ye may be able to withstand in the evil day, and having done all, to stand. Stand therefore, having your loins girt about with truth, and having on the breastplate of righteousness; and your feet shod with the preparation of the gospel of peace; Above all, taking the shield of faith, wherewith ye shall be able to quench all the fiery darts of the wicked. And take the helmet of salvation, and the sword of the Spirit, which is the word of God: Praying always with all prayer and supplication in the Spirit, and watching thereunto with all perseverance and supplication for all saints."

We need to help people think in realistic terms about themselves, and about everything and everyone around them. For example, don't expect too much of yourself or of others. Don't set yourself up for failure, then become depressed when you can't meet such high expectations of yourself. Accept yourself as you are, like Jesus does. He loves you in spite of a failure or the lack of apparent success.

To change our feelings, we must change our thinking. As this is accomplished, then our actions change. You cannot run away from situations, life's stresses, or unsatisfactory conditions. You <u>can</u> change the way you react to them, however, and in this way, you can change your world or environment. <u>You</u> have control. It is up to you to make the changes.

From the points of emphasis in this chapter, you see that you <u>can</u> hang up this Hang-up.

HANG-UP NUMBER FOUR:
Anger

You don't have to live very long before you encounter angry people. You certainly do not counsel many people before you find some that are angry. Anger varies in its intensity and duration. It may start early in childhood with rejection, or it can begin as a result of abuse. Anger can lead to bitterness and unforgiveness that burn deep within to cause lifelong problems until we are freed from its grip. Anger can make it very difficult to relate to others on an intimate level, leading to much frustration in our interpersonal relationships. It can paralyze our ability to respond in an appropriate manner to any given situation.

Anger can be the gateway that Satan uses to oppress us by fears, guilt, rationalization and isolation from others. Satan, our spiritual enemy, can use all of these feelings to aggravate and destroy us.

Anger can also be constructive however, as it can motivate and drive us toward success; impel us toward correcting injustices; or help us to think in a creative manner.

WHAT CAUSES ANGER?
Someone has said that anger is a reaction of indignation in response to another person or situation. There probably are as many causes of anger as there are different situations that we find frustrating. Let us look at some of the causes.

Frustration
Several years ago, Yale University investigators said that anger and aggression arise primarily as a response to frustration. Do you remember the last time you were frustrated by a particular turn of events? Made

you angry, didn't it? Anytime we set our minds on a goal and are continually frustrated in reaching it, we become angry. As frustrations increase, our potential for anger also increases.

Injustice

How often have we gotten angry because of someone's unjust action? Consider Jesus when he drove the money changers out of the temple. He was angry because of the wrong being done and because people were being treated unjustly. Why do you suppose that so many people can get a following? It is because they point out an injustice and start a campaign against the situation with which we can readily identify.

Rejection

We get angry when we are made aware of our own imperfections because this awareness is perceived as a threat that is too big for us to cope with. We are also threatened when there is a challenge to our self-esteem and self-worth. We get angry when we are rejected, put-down, belittled, humiliated, or unjustly criticized. We often try to direct attention toward someone else in an effort to hide our anger, hurt or the threat that we feel.

Learned Response

Children are often brought up in surroundings where there is anger and/or violence, or where family members relate to each other in a very aggressive manner. It may be that verbal communication is always loud and aggressive. These children learn to communicate by responding in a loud, angry manner to frustrations, unpleasant surroundings, or others' actions.

HOW DO WE DEAL WITH ANGER?

The first step is to admit that we are angry. If we continue to deny that we are angry, we will never be able to eliminate anger and its negative effects from our lives.

The next step is to consider the source of our anger. Where does it come from? Why am I angry? Is my anger justified? Should I feel inferior? Is the offense or situation worth all the energy I am putting into being angry? In one year's time will the problem that is making me angry matter?

For example, have you ever had the experience of walking down the street and someone ran into you and almost knocked you down? Anger arose immediately. You turned around and found that the guilty person was blind. What was your response then? The anger seemed to flee quickly. What happened to it? Becoming angry in this situation was your reaction. This example shows that we <u>can</u> control anger.

FACTORS THAT DETERMINE RESPONSES TO ANGER-PRODUCING SITUATIONS

What determines our reaction to anger? No two people respond the same way to an anger-producing situation. Some of the factors that determine our responses are:

Modeling by Parents

Parental modeling of behavior under anger-producing circumstances tends to set our behavior for us. If parents are loud and explosive, then their children tend to be the same way. If parents express anger mildly, their children follow this example.

Socioeconomic Status And Positioning in the Family

These factors apparently play a part in a person's ability to control anger. For example, children from families of lower socioeconomic status, only children and the youngest child in a large family seem to express anger more openly and more violently.

Immaturity

As a person matures, his reactions to frustration and anger become less frequent and more controlled.

Personality Make- up

Some people seem to be more sensitive to frustration and feelings of injustice and are less able to control their reactions to these stresses.

Perception

No two people perceive any given situation alike. Thus, one person gets angry while another person is hardly visibly upset.

WAYS THAT PEOPLE COPE WITH ANGER

What are some commonly observed ways that people cope with anger?

Shifting Responsibility

This is done by blaming others or "kicking the cat."

Avoidance
You practice avoidance by removing yourself from exposure to the anger-producing event or circumstance, or you plunge into some other activity. For example, some people try to hide in alcohol or drugs.

Denial
Pushing anger down inside oneself and not allowing it to show is denial. It is difficult to contain anger or rage inside. Doing so usually brings physical symptoms such as headaches, ulcers, hypertension, heart attacks or psychological reactions such as anxiety, fear, tension and depression. In addition, denial can bring spiritual struggles with bitterness, unforgiveness, or wrath.

Confrontation
Confronting the source of anger and frustration can bring about some of the negative conditions mentioned above. Hopefully, the confrontation will be positive and result in reducing anger and restoring harmony to the situation or relationship.

Religious Experience
A person's religious experience can play a part in his reaction to anger. The Bible deals with the subject of anger very extensively. Anger's various causes are outlined—many are justifiable and many are not. Any good Bible Cyclopedia index or concordance will list these causes. I suggest you study them.

The Bible describes very simply what the Christian's attitude should be toward anger:
1. To be slow in -- **Proverbs 14:17**
2. Not to sin in -- **Ephesians 4:26** and
3. To put away -- **Ephesians 4:31**.

43

Physical or psychological symptoms or other problems such as unforgiveness, bitterness, slander or wrath have to be dealt with. These areas too can be the doorway for Satan and his oppressing forces to move in on you. Be aware of these results and seek the guidance of the Holy Spirit, the Word of God and a Christian counselor, if necessary, in dealing with anger.

Whatever it takes to accomplish it—we need to hang up this hang-up.

HANG-UP NUMBER FIVE:
Fear

Webster's dictionary defines fear as dread, apprehension and alarm. Can you recall the last time you experienced fear? What was it like? Was it pleasant or unpleasant? Your pulse rate increased; you had an empty or peculiar sensation in your stomach. Your mind raced like a computer in considering all the ways you could get away from the situation. Maybe your extremities shook or you were unable to speak. As you can see, physical changes are brought about by fear as we prepare for flight or fight—whatever may be appropriate.

Fear is a very powerful emotion. It can be helpful in small quantities but extreme states of fear can alter the function of many of the organs of our bodies. If this altered function continues over a period of time, or occurs erratically or spasmodically, then it can lead to disease.

TYPES OF FEAR

There are many types of fear: for example, fear of failure, fear of people, fear of disease, fear of open spaces or fear of airplanes.

CAUSES OF FEAR

Fear is a symptom, not a disease. It is usually part of a symptom complex and indicates an underlying psychiatric, emotional or spiritual disturbance.

We are programmed to be fearful by the media and our speech. Our speech is negative. "It scared me to death." "I'd rather die than…." "It's the cold and flu season so I believe I'm getting…." We promote fear by what we say and by what we believe.

THE BIBLE AND FEAR

II Timothy 1:7 says, "For God hath not given us the spirit of fear, but of power, and of love, and of a sound mind." If God does not give fear, then, who does? The devil! God gives us

    1. The spirit of power—The Holy Spirit.

    2. The spirit of love—Jesus, God's son.

You have a sound mind when Jesus and the Holy Spirit abide in you.

I John 4:18 says, "There is no fear in love, but perfect love casteth out fear." The Amplified Bible reads, "There is no fear in love—dread does not exist; but full-grown complete (perfect) love turns fear out of doors and expels every trace of terror!"

We have discovered some antidotes for fear:

    1. the Holy Spirit

    2. Jesus, the spirit of love

    3. the Word of God.

> God's Word perfected in us brings forth love as faith in the Word operates. The more we fill our hearts and minds with the Word, the less fear we have because we are freed from being fearful. The Bible says, "If we know the truth, the truth will make us free." In this instance, knowing the truth frees us from fear.

    4. the anointing.

Isaiah 10:27 says, "And the yoke shall be destroyed because of the anointing." It is that supernatural energizing, driving force within that makes the spirit-filled life forcible, effective and productive in Christian service. If you have received the anointing and it abides in you, then that anointing breaks the yoke of fear.

FEAR AS A SPIRITUAL FORCE

Some people regard fear as a spiritual force just as real and powerful as faith. In this sense, fear would be regarded as the "flip-side" of faith. Faith in action brings a response from our heavenly Father. Fear is believing for the negative. Fear activates Satan and his evil forces.

We can break the power of this spiritual force by having faith in God's Word; praying in the spirit; and using the name of Jesus. We simply take authority over fear in the Name of Jesus, casting it down and casting it out. Again, the Bible says, "Perfect love casts out fear" (I John 4:18). Jesus is that perfect love. Isaiah 59:19 says, "When the enemy shall come in like a flood the Spirit of the Lord shall lift up a standard against him."

Since fear is such a powerful spiritual force, it takes a tremendously powerful counterforce to repel it—the power of the Holy Ghost working in us. This force is available to us today. We have to decide, by an act of our will, to trust God. We have to put our faith in God and His Word rather than in circumstances or our own ability or anything else. We can come against this spiritual force with the Word of God and defeat it. We must take authority over fear and in Jesus' name cast it out.

You can be free from this Hang-up. God's Word provides for your freedom.

HANG-UP NUMBER SIX:
Problems in Marriage and the Family

The family is under attack today as never before. If I made a list of all of the enemies of the family, it would be a very long one. Let's look at the major ones.

SATANIC ATTACK

It appears that Satan has let loose all the forces of hell against the family. I cannot recall a time nor have I read of one in which there was a greater assault against the family. What are some of the devices that Satan uses? Let's list these as well.

Divorce

Did you know that divorce ends one of every two marriages today? There are many devices that Satan uses to bring about divorce: for example, alcoholism, drugs, sexual incompatibility, or unfaithfulness by a spouse. Emotional immaturity in one or both partners is another big cause, as are irresponsibility, selfishness, and the inability to be intimate.

God hates divorce. Notice—I didn't say that God hates divorcees or the parties to a divorce. I said, "He hates divorce." Why? Because God instituted and ordained marriage, the home, children and the family. This is the norm for man. This is the way God created man—to be married to a woman. It was Adam and Eve, not Adam and Steve. Marriage is figurative of God's union with the church.

Historically, marriage has been the cornerstone of the family. Happily married people do a better job of rearing children. All of today's "happy marrieds" were not always so, but they worked at it. Today, divorce is easy; some states allow no fault divorces.

Too often divorce leaves a scar on children. Separation of the child from one of the parents he loves can leave emotional and psychic scars. These scars can lead to an excessive emotional vulnerability, making it much more difficult for the child to cope with the normal stresses of life. It also makes it difficult to trust and love within that child's own family unit once he or she grows up.

<u>Secular Humanism</u>

The second big device Satan uses is Secular Humanism. This doctrine is an attempt by man to find the answers for all of life's questions within himself. It puts the self up to be worshiped instead of God. Secular Humanism teaches a one-world view of man, big government, situation ethics, and no God, salvation, or eternity.

THE PUBLIC SCHOOL SYSTEM

Another enemy of the family is the public school system. By and large, our public school systems are controlled by Secular Humanists. Humanism is taught and God is denied. More and more, humanists are trying to claim that children belong to the state instead of their parents and, therefore, must be taught by the state. Does this sound like Russia? You're right—it does. Can you believe it is really happening right here in America? Well, it is. We had better start doing something about this situation before it is too late.

TELEVISION

Another enemy of the family is television. Most children watch 30-50 hours of television per week. Over the course of a lifetime, this can equal 320,000 commercials. Some families use the television as a baby sitter. You should know what goes into your child's mind. Remember, "As the twig is bent, so grows the tree."

THE MEDIA
Low moral standards, the desire for sensationalism and the mania to sell papers and magazines make much of what your child reads unfit for human consumption.

FEMINISM
The desire of the feminist is to destroy the family as we know it today. Can we allow that to happen?

MATERIALISM
Families are programmed, by so much of what they see and learn, to think of materialism as success. Success is not things. This kind of success will not satisfy.

PORNOGRAPHY AND VIOLENCE
The television screens are full of porn and violence. There are very, very few family programs anymore. It seems that the more violent the programming is, the more sex, nudity and profanity that are displayed, the greater the ratings of particular shows.

DRUGS AND ALCOHOL
More than ever before, the young people in our society are accepting alcohol as a ready alternative to drugs. It is a form of escapism for people of all ages.

ROCK MUSIC
Rock music is habituating, if not addictive. When a group of young people visited Africa and performed their rock music, the natives asked them, "Why do you call the demons?" The beat of the music, they said, called up demon spirits. These natives could not understand why these young people would play this type of music since they professed to be Christians.

HOMOSEXUALITY

Homosexuality is on the rise and is being accepted as an alternate life style. God puts a curse on those who practice this lifestyle. Remember: It was Adam and Eve, not Adam and Steve.

MOBILITY

America has become a country of people on the move. One study says that the average American family moves at least five times every two years. Another study shows that 20% of all families move more than 100 miles each year. **Mobility destroys stability, roots and relationships. It destroys families.**

God is on the side of those who stand up for marriage and the family. If God be for us, who can be against us? Knowing who our enemy is can play a big part in obtaining the victory over our enemies. Too often we have found that the enemy is us.

ATTRIBUTES PRESENT IN GOOD MARRIAGES

We have talked about some of the enemies of marriage and the family. Let's look at some of the things that are important in making marriages work, those factors that make bad marriages good and good marriages better.

Commitment

There must be a commitment by each party to make the marriage work. This is a decision of the will that we have to make if our marriages are to succeed and last. Are you committed to your mate?

<u>Love</u>

There must be love. **Ephesians 5:25** says that a husband should "agape" his wife. Agape love is defined as love that is by choice, not by feeling. Agape love is love that chooses to do the highest good for the wife in spite of her response. In other words, the wife's response to the husband's actions makes no difference in his choice to do the right thing. Agape love gives without expecting a return. If you give you will receive. By the same token, the wife is to "philandros" her husband. This instruction is found in **Titus 2:4.** Philandros means that the wife is to constantly be her husband's best friend, his admirer. Perhaps "encourager" is the word that best describes what a wife should be to her husband.

It is written that when God made woman to be man's companion, He didn't make her from man's head to rule over him. She was not made from man's feet to be trampled by him. She was made from a rib taken from his side to be equal with him, from under his arm to be protected by him, and from near his heart to be loved by him.

Let us never lose sight of the goal of loving and fulfilling one another in our marriages. That is what life is all about.

<u>Communication</u>

Next, there should be communication between the marriage partners. Communication should be a two-way system that each understands and participates in. Communication includes being able to communicate effectively, negotiating, and balancing partners' differences.

<u>Trust</u>

Another essential is trust. If you don't trust

your mate, why did you marry? If you trust, you are not jealous.

<u>Responsibility</u>

Being a responsible person is another essential ingredient in the successful marriage. Not only must you find the right person, you must be the right person.

<u>Gifts, Goals and God</u>

Dr. James E. Kilgore says that marriages need gifts, goals and God. He expands on this theme by saying, "We need to remember our mates occasionally with gifts but the greatest gift we can give is ourselves."

The gift of sharing

We should share ourselves with our mates. Spend quality time together.

Goals

Just as gifts are important, so are goals. There is no place for competition in marriage as it destroys relationships. All of us have a basic need to share with someone else. This can find its greatest expression and satisfaction in a happy marriage relationship.

The absence of shared goals can create an emptiness that nothing else can fill. We cannot afford to build individual worlds for ourselves as they separate us. Our goals and dreams in marriage only come true when they are shared.

God

Every marriage can be a greater marriage if God is included in it—if each partner has a vital, living relationship with God the Father, Jesus the Son and the Holy Spirit. We cannot depend on ritual; our relationship must be personal. We must worship together as well as pray together. A family altar should be established in every home as soon as a couple is married and should become an institution for that family. There should be times of family prayer, worship, and teaching. We need to give our children a strong faith in God to live by. We can do this best by being an example. The closer we get to God, the closer we get to each other.

God likens marriage to Christ's relationship with the church. I believe this is indicative of the importance that God places on marriage and the family.

CHILD REARING
Child rearing is one of the most important tasks we will ever undertake; yet, we have no experience or training in it. As parents, we have roles and responsibilities thrust on us for which we are ill-prepared. Just about every vocation you can name requires education and training to fit a person to the task. This education and training varies from a few months to several years, depending on the particular vocation. In contrast, the job of child rearing has virtually no training for it. Much of what we think we know about parenting comes from our experiences with our parents—which may be good or bad. What do we parents do? Most of us wind up reading books on the subject, or we do what comes naturally, or we give up in despair.

The Bible offers some guidance and help in child rearing. You will find scriptures that can be divided into two kinds: comments about children and comments about parents and parenting. There are scriptures on parental duties such as:

    1. teaching -- **Deuteronomy 6:6-7**
    2. training -- **Proverbs 22:6**

3. providing for -- **II Corinthians 12:14**
4. nurturing—**Ephesians 6:4** and **Colossians 3:21**
5. controlling—**I Timothy 3:4**
6. loving—**Titus 2:4.**

There are other scriptures that speak about the correction of children: **Proverbs 13:24; 19:18; 22:15; 23:13 and 29:15 and 17.**

There are special promises to children:
1. reverent children -- **Deuteronomy 5:16**
2. forsaken children -- **Psalm 27:10**
3. early seekers -- **Proverbs 8:17**
4. obedient children -- **Proverbs 8:32**
5. little children—**Mark 10:14**
6. the commandment with promise -- **Ephesians 6:1-3**.

There are very few directives in the Bible on child rearing as specific directions are not there. **Deuteronomy 6:1-8** puts together many of the principles for us and gives an overview of Christian child rearing. Even though these principles were written to the early Israelites, they are very practical and relevant to modern child rearing and parenting. The following passage is the Amplified Bible's version of **Deuteronomy 6:1-8:**

> Now this is the instruction, the laws, and the precepts, which the Lord your God commanded me to teach you, that you might do them in the land to which you go to possess it; That you may (reverently) fear the Lord your God, you and your son and your son's son, and keep all His statutes and His commandments, which I command you, all the days of your life; and that your days may be prolonged. Hear therefore, O Israel, and be watchful to do them; that it may be well with you, and that you may increase exceedingly as the Lord God of your

fathers has promised you, in a land flowing
with milk and honey. Hear, O Israel: the Lord
our God is one Lord—the only Lord. And you
shall love the Lord your God with all your
[mind and] heart, and with your entire being,
and with all your might. And these words,
which I am commanding you this day shall be
[first] in your *own* mind *and* heart; [then] You
shall whet and sharpen them, so as to make
them penetrate, and teach *and* impress them
diligently upon the [minds and] hearts of your
children, and shall talk of them when you sit
in your house, and when you walk by the way,
and when you lie down and when you rise up.
And you shall bind them as a sign upon your
hand, and they shall be as frontlets (forehead
bands) between your eyes.

ATTRIBUTES OF CHRISTIAN PARENTING

Christian parenting involves several things:

1. Listening -- Good parents seek to hear God's
commandments and to understand them so well that they
are written on the tables of their hearts. The commandments
are evidenced in their lives; they are a part of their being.
This depth of knowledge comes only through regular
study and application of God's Word as it is interpreted
by the Holy Spirit.

2. Obeying -- Knowledge of God's Word is not
enough. In addition to hearing and knowing, we must
obey by doing what God has commanded. When we, as
parents, fail to obey God then it is more difficult for our
children to obey God.

3. Loving -- We are to love the Lord and give
ourselves to Him—spirit, soul, and body.

4. Teaching -- Teaching is done four ways:

Diligently -- It is done right and not taken lightly.

Repeatedly -- Teaching children is done repeatedly, over and over, all during the day and night.

Naturally -- We should look for teaching opportunities in whatever we are doing—regardless of whether it is done when we are sitting, lying down, going out, or coming in.

Personally -- Parents should strive to provide a model for whatever is being said or taught in the home. The most significant teaching, the teaching that is most effective, is teaching that is done in the home by example.

CHILD REARING PROBLEMS

When you are having problems in child rearing, recognize that there are some common causes:

1. Unstable home conditions --When parents are not getting along well, the child feels anxious, guilty, angry. Anxious because he is fearful that the home is threatened; guilty for he fears that he is the cause of the problem; angry because he feels left out, forgotten, ignored. Sometimes the child may feel manipulated into taking sides. Fear of abandonment is the greatest fear of children.

2. Failure of parents --This may consist of physical or psychological abuse. The child is rejected, nagged, unloved or spasmodically rejected and loved, and given inconsistent discipline. Children will often show disruptive behavior when these conditions exist in the home. This, in turn, usually angers or annoys the parents.

3. Needs that are not met -- Some of those unmet needs might be for security, acceptance, significance, love, praise, discipline and a need for God. Failure to meet these needs most often leads to immaturity, resulting in lifelong problems for the child involved.

4. Neglect of spiritual life and of the child -- **(Psalm 78:1-8).** We should follow the scriptural admonition in **II Peter 1:5:** "Add to your faith, virtue; and to virtue knowledge." Give your children a dynamic faith in God with which to live. Add solid teaching on virtue so they know the importance God places on this characteristic. Then give them knowledge and an education.

5. Poor Communication -- Communication is an absolute necessity among family members. Good communication leads to good interpersonal relationships among family members. Good interpersonal relations start with Jesus Christ. As believers, we need to apply the principles of love as noted in **I Corinthians 13**— following them will develop good interpersonal relations within the family. Good communication and interpersonal relations require determination, effort and skill.

Poor communication gives rise to physical effects such as fatigue, strain, headaches, stomach upsets and ulcers, and can trigger almost every human emotion.

Good communication is vital in marriage and family relationships as well as in child rearing.

6. Life Experiences -- Some other causes that should be noted are sickness, handicaps, death of an important person, traumatic early experiences, peer rejection, and experiences of failure. All of these situations can create problems in later life.

Most children grow up normally in spite of parental mistakes or failures. Poor homes don't always translate into problem children. As you can see from the list above, oftentimes problems arise which are independent of parental action.

BEHAVIOR MANAGEMENT

The most common method used to manage unacceptable behavior is physical punishment. If it is used too often however, it will not do any good. There are times when punishment is in order and the Bible sanctions using it during those times.

There are other forms of discipline that are good and need to be used. We should train our children by rewarding good behavior. If we speak the Word of God over our children from infancy, if we emphasize the positive by telling them how they belong to God, how they are good children, how they are smart and capable, then we can mold them in a very positive way. Pray with your children. Pray over them every day, claiming God's best for them, and they will thrive spiritually and behaviorally. Program your children's minds positively. Let them know that Jesus loves them, is watching over them and is interested in everything they do.

Pray in the spirit for your children. Take dominion over Satan and bind his influence over your children. Put a hedge of prayer and the power of the anointing of God around them daily.

When you correct your children, take the time to teach them also. Read the Word of God to them. Show them where God gives you the responsibility of rearing them and how they are instructed to obey you. Let them know that God instructs this way because God loves them. Let them know that you are carrying out God's plan because you love both God and them. Pray with your children after you have corrected them. Ask God's forgiveness and thank Him for His care of your family.

Never be too proud or hung up to admit to your children that you were wrong and to ask them to forgive you. They will forgive you and you can go forward from there.

I am not trying to cover the entire subject of child rearing in this chapter as there are many references that give great counsel on this subject. What I have given are some basic guidelines and attitudinal directions that I believe are very important in rearing children.

Here are "Twelve Rules for Raising a Delinquent."

Twelve Rules for Raising a Delinquent

1. Begin with infancy to give the child everything he wants. In this way he will grow up to believe the world owes him a living.

2. When he picks up bad words laugh at him. This will make him think he is cute. It will also encourage him to pick up "cuter phrases."

3. Never give him any spiritual training. Wait till he is 21 and let him decide for himself.

4. Avoid the use of the word wrong. It could cause a guilt complex to develop in him. This will condition him to believe later when he is arrested for stealing a car, that society is against him and he is being punished.

5. Pick up everything he leaves lying around, books, shoes, clothing. Do everything for him so he will be experienced in throwing all responsibility on to others.

6. Let him read any printed matter he can get his hands on. Be careful that the silverware and drinking glasses are sterilized but let his mind feed on garbage.

7. Quarrel frequently in the presence of your children. In this way they will not be too shocked when the house is broken up.

8. Give the child all the spending money he wants. Never let him earn his own. Why should he have things as tough as you had them?

9. Satisfy his every craving for food, drink, comfort. See that every sensual desire is gratified. Denial may lead to frustration.

10. Take his part against teachers, neighbors, and

policemen. They are all prejudiced against your child.

11. When he gets into real trouble apologize for yourself by saying, "I never could do anything with him."

12. Prepare for a life of grief, you will be apt to have it.

Note:These rules were developed by the Houston, Texas Police Department

HANG-UP NUMBER SEVEN:
Marital Conflict

Many problems arise in families. Almost one out of two marriages today ends in divorce. As you move about in any part of our society, you encounter many people who have gone through divorce. It seems that divorce is almost universal.

Marital conflict comes in spite of "being in love." When you talk to people before they marry, you hear "But our love will be different. We can overcome all kinds of obstacles." These couples can overcome many things, but emotional immaturity in one or both is very difficult to overcome. This is the one factor most often seen in marriages experiencing conflict.

Another problem, especially among young people, is the prevailing attitude toward marriage. Many young people see no permanence in the marriage relationship; rather, they view divorce as a means to get rid of an undesired mate if the relationship doesn't work. This attitude is in direct contrast to attitudes of couples who married 30-40 years ago. Then the attitude was, "We will make our marriage work. Oh sure, we will have differences, but we will work them out." Divorce was frowned on; it was not socially accepted.

With the increase in the divorce rate, we see the change in attitudes and thinking about marriage. It is regarded very lightly, more like a temporary arrangement. There is little of the feeling my generation had that a union created by God is permanent. That part of the marriage ceremony "What God has joined together, let no man put asunder" has been forgotten, tossed out of the window.

CAUSES OF MARITAL CONFLICT

Emotional Immaturity

One of the most frequent causes of marital conflict I have seen is emotional immaturity in one or both partners. Along with this problem are other issues caused by selfishness, self-centeredness, exorbitant demands for attention, and a desire to control the partner.

Failure to Become "One"

Another problem often seen is shown in Genesis where God tells us that after a man gets married, he and his wife should leave and cleave. They should leave their parents' home and cleave to each other. Nosy, interfering parents who are either trying to control their married children, or who seek vicarious pleasure through their children's marriages should back off and go do their own thing, leaving "the kids" alone. Failure to follow God's direct command on this issue will bring heartache, separation, and despair to a young couple. It can likely be the disturbing influence that causes the marriage to end in divorce.

According to *Strong's Concordance,* the Hebrew word for cleave means to stick, to adhere, to be joined together. It implies that the union is inseparable: The husband and wife can't separated into two parts as they are one. They share in loving, in each other's differences, in each other's desires, goals and problems. Being one includes sex and the physical side of life together—but there is far more than that. Being one also means sharing successes, failures, joys, hopes and defeats. We remain uniquely ourselves, yet we are one.

Sex

Most couples have some sexual problems in their marriage. Sexual difficulties can cause other problems, or the stress and tension of other problems can make it difficult to fulfill the sexual role in marriage, leading to other problems. Husbands—Be loving, kind and tender toward your wives and always considerate of them. **Wives—Do not, I repeat, do not use sex as an agent to bargain with or as a bribe for desired favors or actions.**

Paul, in his writings to the Corinthians, gives very explicit instructions to married couples about their sexual adaptation to each other. Heed Paul's advice. He shows us how to deal with the added stress of passion: Get married is his admonition.

I have always been amazed by people—how we can be so in love before marriage, doing everything we can to please each other, yet shortly after the marriage, we are at odds with one another.

Often this conflict is about sex. We forget that God made sex. He made it to be fun and pleasurable as well as a way to reproduce our kind. Satan has perverted sex. He has made it something that is earthy, dirty, animalistic and debased. God meant sex to be something that is uplifting, that makes us one, that fulfills and satisfies. He meant for it to be an experience that is physical and spiritual.

As marriage partners, we must remain mindful of our mates' needs as well as our own. Sex must not be allowed to become a battleground or a bargaining instrument.

Money

This is another frequent cause of marital conflict. The management of money is not a talent shared by everyone alike. If money management is a problem, then get some counseling on how to handle your finances. The counseling process will also help you to find answers to questions such as Who handles the checkbook? Whose money is it? Who makes the financial decisions? What things are needed and what are desirable? Do we need a budget? How much should we give to the church? What happens if there is a shortage of money?

Non-communication

So many marriages start off great but soon go very sour because of the lack of communication. It is absolutely essential that you and your spouse be on the same wavelength and communicate effectively. Husbands—You need to say these three little words—"I love you"—every day. Wives—Remember to be affectionate and say "I love you" often, too.

Religion

I cannot stress this aspect too much. Do not be unequally yoked with an unbeliever. Do not be unequally yoked with someone of a different faith without first having a thorough understanding of each other's faith, without discussing at great length your differences in religious beliefs and how you plan to manage them. Seek counsel from your pastoral staff and deal with your differences before marriage.

Values

What are yours? What are your betrothed's? How do they differ? How are they alike? These differences should be settled before marriage or there is great potential for conflict. Ask yourself these questions: How do you feel about using credit cards? What part the church should play in your life? What things are of major importance to you? Should wives work? Is television good or bad? Is divorce right or wrong?

Values that we have been taught or are very dear to us can be grounds for conflict. If our values are attacked, then we defend them. Conflict arises and away we go.

Stress from Sources Outside the Home

Stress from sources outside the home can cause marital conflict. Some of these outside stress factors are

1. Nagging in-laws that criticize or make inordinate demands

2. Children -- interference by children in their parents' affairs or demands by children that tax their parents' ability to comply

3. Friends -- any kind of relationship with a friend that puts stress on the marital relationship

4. Crises that disrupt normal family routine and functioning

5. Vocational demands that put pressure on the husband or wife to perform or succeed

Boredom

Why do so many couples divorce after 25-30 years of marriage? They have reared a family. The kids are gone and mom and dad are left with each other. Often they find themselves living with a stranger—someone they don't know and don't want to know. Everything they do is routine. They have settled into a rut. They get bored. Rather than try to put life into the marriage, the couple divorces.

We spend so much time making money, making friends, or making a life for our family that we forget to make room for them. When we do stop in later life to make room for our family—they are gone. It really isn't worth it. You can have all the things the world says means success, but without love, without someone to share it with, it is only boredom. I repeat: It isn't worth it!

THE EFFECTS OF MARITAL CONFLICT

1. Despair -- Caught in the web of marital conflict and watching as one's marriage disintegrates before your eyes brings despair

2. Confusion -- Facing a lot of conflict and despair may be confusing and cause the partners to wonder, Where do I go next?

3. Withdrawal -- Rather than face the social stigma and devastation of divorce, many couples withdraw in the home and from the marriage. To all outward appearances, everything is OK, but there is no love, no communication, no intimacy in the relationship. The marriage has died on the vine.

4. Abandonment -- It is said that 50,000 American men walk out of their marriages and
disappear every year, creating single-parent homes. When family pressures and marital pressures become too heavy, they leave.

5. Divorce -- This avenue is becoming more and more popular as a way of dealing with conflict in marriage. It is producing couples who have been married more than once, some even four or five times. The likelihood of these people being successful in a marriage relationship is very slim.

MARITAL CONFLICT AND THE BIBLE

There is very little in the Bible about marital conflict. There are some broad-based principles about marriage and the marriage relationship, however. The Bible is very specific in dealing with the attitudes, the beliefs, the sin, and the resulting strife of marital conflicts. Immaturity, selfishness and pride are all dealt with in the scriptures. If we study the Word of God, determine how we measure up, and bring our lives into harmony with the Word, we will avoid marital conflict.

WHAT WE CAN DO ABOUT MARITAL CONFLICT

1. Seek counseling from a godly counselor or pastor. In counseling you can learn how to communicate with each other.

2. Learn how to build your marriage on Biblical principles. Get into the Word of God and see how you measure up. Try **I Corinthians 13** for instance, the "Love Chapter." Measure your love and esteem for your spouse in the light of this scripture.

3. Learn how to solve problems and make decisions.

4. Become aware, and stay aware, of issues and situations in your marriage that can potentially cause conflict. Avoid them.

HOW WE CAN AVOID MARITAL CONFLICT

Biblical principles of marriage need to be taught by the church. Strong families mean strong churches and strong homes. Strong families and homes create a strong nation. Instead of leaving this task up to godless professors and teachers, the church needs to take on this role. The leaders of our churches need to live consistent Christian lives, modeling for our young people the kind of marriages and homes that are successful because they are built on the Word of God.

Christian couples need to submit themselves to

God, order their homes and relationships according to the Word of God, and teach their children these principles.

Our Catholic friends started, and many other churches have followed their example of sponsoring, a Marriage Encounter for married couples in their churches. Marriage Encounter is designed to get couples away from distracting influences for 48-72 hours and teach them about commitment to each other. It is designed to make any marriage better and especially to help poor marriages. If you have the opportunity, get into a Marriage Encounter.

God started marriage with Adam and Eve. Because Adam was lonely, God made him a mate. God wants our marriages to succeed. As Christians, we cannot be effective witnesses when our relationship with our mates isn't strong.

Marriage is the most intimate of human relationships. A good marriage is very satisfying and fulfilling. A bad marriage is misery "gone to seed." We can make the difference between having a good marriage or a bad one by ordering our lives and our marriages according to the Word of God. If God puts the marriage in order, He will bless it.

Husbands—Stand up and be counted for God. Decide to be all that God wants you to be as a husband and a father. Decide to be the priest of your home. Decide to take your rightful place as the head of your house, in the Lord. Put any sin, sexual and otherwise, under the blood. Study God's Word. Learn how you can be the head of your family. Order your life, your family, your marriage according to God's Word. In return, God will richly bless you with a successful marriage and godly children. God will also prosper everything you do.

Marital conflict is a Hang-up that we can do without.

HANG-UP NUMBER EIGHT:
Guilt

In psychiatric jargon guilt is defined as an emotion resulting from doing what is conceived of as wrong, thereby violating superego precepts. Guilt results in feelings of worthlessness and, at times, the need for punishment. Closely associated with guilt is shame. The latter is defined as an emotion resulting from failure to live up to self-expectations.

Our feelings or perception of guilt are closely tied to our background through the teachings we receive as children, our "programming." We are programmed by what our parents teach us and by what we learn growing up. Our minds are taught that we should do, or not do, certain things, how and what to believe, what is good for us, what is bad. If, at some later time, we find our behavior violating what we have been taught or led to believe by our upbringing, then we tend to feel guilty. We feel that we have done wrong. This in itself detracts from our self-worth. We feel ourselves to be of less value because we have transgressed; we have failed. If we continue to do whatever it is that makes us feel guilty, then we can find ourselves feeling worthless.

If we have been taught that when we do something that is wrong we receive punishment (and most of us have been taught this), we naturally feel that wrongdoing on our part has to be "paid for" by suffering punishment. This allows us to deal with our feelings of guilt. If we have paid our "dues" we can forgive ourselves and stop feeling guilty. We regain our self-worth. There is only one thing wrong with this approach, however. We don't usually deal with our guilt feelings this simply. We excuse ourselves with all kinds of reasons. Here are some of them:

1. We blame others.

2. We attribute our behavior to circumstances.

3. We rationalize that it was for a good cause.

4. We whitewash the guilt with good intentions or motivations.

5. We shove the guilt down inside us and deny that it exists, or cover it up.

6. We may try to drown our guilt feelings in drink or drugs.

If guilt is not dealt with in a realistic manner that will resolve or remove its feelings, then it can lead to depression, withdrawal or suicide.

Guilt can be divided into various types such as

1. Legal guilt -- This occurs when one breaks a law.

2. Social guilt -- This occurs when one breaks social laws of behavior and therefore feels shame, remorse or disgrace.

3. Moral guilt -- This occurs when we violate our conscience or personal standards of right and wrong.

4. Religious or theological guilt -- When we knowingly violate God's laws, this is referred to in the Bible as sin. The Bible teaches that there is forgiveness when we sin, if we will seek it.

HOW THE BIBLE TREATS GUILT

The Bible does not use guilt as a motivation to do good. To the contrary, the Bible teaches forgiveness. This is a major theme of scripture. Jesus Christ came to save sinners; He came to forgive; He came to lift up—not push down.

In his writings, Paul talks about how godly sorrow brings forgiveness and restoration. Guilt offers torment that can be relieved only by penance—which is impossible. Satan deceives many into trying this method. They find, however, that it doesn't work.

Dr. Clyde Narramore talks about "constructive sorrow" which leads to "constructive change." Release from guilt comes when we realize that we have broken God's law or sinned; repent and change our direction by moving toward God rather than away from Him; ask God to forgive us; and accept His forgiveness.

This process is outlined in the following scriptures:

Numbers 32:23

"Behold ye have sinned against the Lord; and be sure your sin will find you out."

David, a man after God's own heart, is a good example for us. When he sinned against God, he acknowledged that his sin (guilt) was ever before him. Day and night David felt God's hand upon him. When he kept silent and did not confess his sin, even his "bones waxed old." When David humbled himself, acknowledged his sin, and sought and received the Lord's forgiveness, he then could say, "I waited patiently for God to help me; then he listened and heard my cry. He lifted me out of the pit of despair, out from the bog and the mire, and set my feet on a hard firm path and steadied me as I walked along. He has given me a new song to sing, of praises to our God. Now many will hear of the glorious things he did for me and stand in awe before the Lord, and put their trust in Him" **Psalm 40: 1-3.**

Psalm 86:5

> "For thou, Lord, art good and ready to forgive; and plenteous in mercy unto all them that call upon thee."

Proverbs 28:13

> "He that covereth his sins shall not prosper; but whoso confesseth and forsaketh them shall have mercy."

I John 1:9

> "If we confess our sins, he is faithful and just to forgive us our sins, and to cleanse us from all unrighteousness."

As you can see, guilt and sin are directly tied to forgiveness and the promise that if we will forsake our sin and turn to Him, then God will respond by forgiving. We no longer feel guilty or are conscious of our sin when we are forgiven.

Many well-meaning people (preachers, among them) who are motivated to help others, try to do so by putting a guilt trip on those they are helping. The Bible does not do that. Jesus didn't, either. When the young woman who was caught in the act of adultery was brought to him, he did not accuse her or put guilt on her. Jesus forgave her, loved her, and warned her to "go and sin no more."

If you repeat the sin, then the guilt will return. You must change and forsake the sin. **Romans 4:7** says, "Blessed are they whose iniquities are forgiven, and whose sins are covered." Romans 8:1 says, "There is therefore now no condemnation to them which are in Christ Jesus, who walk not after the flesh, but after the Spirit."

There is another aspect to forgiveness that must be mentioned: We must forgive others if we are to receive

God's forgiveness. **Matthew 6:14-15** says, "For if ye forgive men their trespasses, your heavenly Father will also forgive you. But if ye forgive not men their trespasses, neither will your Father forgive your trespasses." In other words, if we forgive, then we will be forgiven.

THE CAUSES OF GUILT
Many things can cause guilt. Here are some of them.

How We Are Taught
Our self-concept is greatly influenced by our own family. If we are warm, loving, caring, forgiving and accepting of our children, then they will not feel guilt. If there is strife between the parents or if they fuss and blame others, then they can cause feelings of guilt in their children. Many situations in the home cause feelings of shame and these feelings are translated into guilt.

Feelings of Inferiority
In his book *Guilt and Grace,* Paul Torneier says there is no delineation between guilt and inferiority: In other words, if you feel inferior then you translate that feeling into guilt. Many people feel inferior or have poor self-worth. I remember my own experience as a teenager and young man. During those times I felt a lot of guilt. The guilt in my case, however, was actually a feeling of inferiority.

Satan
If Satan can slip an oppressive spirit of poor self-worth, poor self-image or guilt into our surroundings to harass and trouble us, he will do it.

Social Pressures
These play a role in feelings of shame or inferiority that we translate into feelings of guilt. Young people

are surrounded by peer pressure to conform or to fulfill certain expectations. Often the latter is helped along by unrealistically high hopes from parents. Many times parents try to live vicariously through their children and thus pressure their children to produce or play roles unsuited for them.

Faulty Development of Conscience

Conscience development varies widely among people. Beginning with Freud, psychologists and psychiatrists have claimed that our conscience is molded early in life by the attitudes, teachings, expectations and prohibitions of our parents. Freud claimed that children learn how to act in order to avoid punishment. Those parents who are good role models provide a home that is warm, loving, accepting, predictable and secure. There is more emphasis on approval and encouragement and less emphasis on punishment and criticism. A child raised in those surroundings knows he is loved when he is bad and when he is good. This child experiences forgiveness.

On the other side of the coin, however, are children who have poor role models in their parents. The homes in which they raised are places where much is demanded of them. Criticism is frequent, and the prevailing attitude is punitive. These surroundings produce anger in the child—which, in turn, brings rebellion and guilt. Often the child has a sense of little worth and guilt.

Proper parental instruction, given in an atmosphere of love and encouragement, can instill moral values and ideals in young people and provide a foundation for the growth and development of godliness. This type of grounding gives a person the freedom to compare the world against Christian ideals and make a choice to follow the Lord Jesus Christ.

When Biblical teaching is provided in an honest,

open atmosphere of inquiry for truth and appraisal of experience, then a level of personal growth and maturity occurs that would never be possible otherwise. On the other hand, if we are trained to think in a very rigid manner about right and wrong, if we are convinced of our own imperfections and incompetence, if we are fearful of failure or punishment and lack an awareness of God's love and forgiveness, then we will be plagued with feelings of inferiority, poor self-esteem and guilt.

Paul's epistles emphasize forgiving one another. If I am to believe Paul's writings (and I do), then God wants us to be free from guilt.

Through His sacrifice and His Word, God has provided a way for us to be free of this Hang-up.

HANG-UP NUMBER NINE:
Poor Interpersonal Relations

This is one of the most important subjects in this book. All of life is centered around interpersonal relationships, whether satisfying or not. When God created us, He saw that it was not good for man to be alone. God saw how lonely Adam was. and that the relationships with animals were not satisfying or sufficient to meet his needs. So, God created woman—the man with the womb. He created Eve and brought her to the man. (Of course, Adam was smitten right away.) Thus began interpersonal relationships—with the first man and the first woman. As Adam and Eve enlarged their family and the world expanded, then there was a greater need for interpersonal relationships. These relations can be smooth, supportive and characterized by clean communication, or they can be strained and conflicted.

Harry Stack Sullivan, an early American psychiatrist, maintained that all personal growth and healing, as well as all personal conflict and regression, come through relationships with others.

What does the Bible teach about interpersonal relationships? Let's look at two familiar scripture passages. First is the Golden Rule. Its basis is interpersonal relationships: "Do unto others as you would have them do unto you." This instruction is uncomplicated and to the point. It doesn't say, "Get the other guy before he gets you." Nor does it say that, "If he treats you OK, then do thus and so." The Golden Rule simply tells us what to do—and to do it regardless of how the other person treats us. The Golden Rule is related to God's law of sowing and reaping: i.e., if we sow good, we reap good.

Second is the Sermon on the Mount. It contains much instruction on how to treat others and it teaches us about peacemaking, loving our enemies, being merciful, judging, and giving.

Jesus Christ is the supreme example of a person with good interpersonal relationships. Why? Because of the great love he had for his fellow man. He demonstrated to us the truths outlined in **I Corinthians 13**, the "Love Chapter." He was driven by God's love—agape. We need to emulate his example, and strive to live like he did. Jesus showed us that the essence of living is giving. In contrast to that, man wants to receive and store up. God's way is to give; and as we give, we receive more from God, our source, and others.

If we are to have good interpersonal relationships, then we start by following the example of the Lord Jesus Christ. We must add to this a determination to develop skills in this important area of our lives. We need to develop good communication skills; be mindful of others; and strive to get along with others. All of these skills are learned behaviors which we can acquire by working on developing them, praying about them, and seeking God's help.

CAUSES OF POOR INTERPERSONAL RELATIONS

What are some of the causes of poor interpersonal relations?

Attitudes, Behaviors and Negative Emotions

1. Attitudes and actions
   Our attitudes toward others combined with our actions can bring strife or peace. We can create conflict and distrust, or we can promote trusting, warm, supportive

relationships with each other.
2. Behavior that demands attention
3. Greed
4. Bitterness
5. Anger
6. Fear (e.g., fear of failure, fear of people, fear of rejection, etc.)
7. Rebellion
8. Prejudice
9. Insecurity
10. Distrust of others
11. Unforgiveness
12. Inability to open up, share or be intimate

Conflict

The world is full of conflict today—interpersonally, socially, politically, economically. Family members are against family members. Conflict is displayed before us in a very graphic manner on our televisions. What is it that we are seeking?

Conflict isn't all bad, however. While it is often destructive and very threatening, conflict can also serve the very useful purpose of classifying goals, unifying a group, or bringing previously ignored disagreements to a point of discussion and resolution.

Conflict should make us stop and ask the question, What is the real issue at hand? It might surprise us to learn how often just asking this question will help to resolve the conflict.

Poor Communication

Communication breakdown stops all interchange between people. No communication leads to no understanding, which leads to no interpersonal relationships. Good communication is absolutely essential to good interpersonal relations.

There are two kinds of communication: verbal and non-verbal. Each affects and colors the other. The sender must send a clear message. The clear message that was sent must be received by the receiver. There can be many slips in this process: We can fail to send a clear message, or we can fail to receive the message, or the message is not clear. Feedback is another important aspect of communication. If two people can communicate, they should be able to level with each other. If the message isn't clear, you can let that be known and the effort can be made to make the message clear so that the message which is sent is, in fact, the message that is received.

Good communication is very satisfying to both the sender and the receiver. It adds fullness and completion to interpersonal relationships like nothing else does. Good communication is part of caring and knowing the other person. It brings intimacy to an otherwise drab relationship.

THE EFFECTS OF POOR INTERPERSONAL RELATIONS

The effects of poor interpersonal relations can be classified as physical, psychological, social, and spiritual.

Physical

Most of us have experienced the physical effects of stress or tension: fatigue, tension, muscle spasms, headaches, indigestion, upset stomach. John Powell wrote, "When I repress my emotions, my stomach keeps score." When we cover our true feelings and try to hide them, we often wind up with these physical effects.

Psychological

Almost every human emotion and corresponding action can be associated with poor interpersonal relations—ranging from uncooperativeness to homicide. When there is tension, we may often feel depressed, shameful, guilty, impotent, or lack self-confidence. As a result of having these feelings, we may not think very clearly and do or say things that we later regret.

Social

The social effects of poor interpersonal relations range from violence on the one hand to complete withdrawal and isolation on the other. It may mean the breakup of a previously very valued and meaningful relationship—such as losing a girlfriend or ending a marriage, business partnership or church affiliation.

Spiritual

Poor interpersonal relations will prevent spiritual growth. When our spiritual growth is stunted, it brings tension between us and God, the Father. Like Adam and Eve, we are separated from God.

We must weigh every aspect of our lives to determine if our attitudes are right. For example, are we being selfish? Is God pleased with what is happening? Do our actions bring glory to Him and His cause?

There are two tables I want to share with you: "The Directions and Tactics in Conflict." and "Guidelines for Communication." Both tables offer very good suggestions on how to negotiate when there is conflict and how to continue to communicate in spite of the conflict. The second table gives guidelines on how to maintain communication. If you practice what these tables suggest, you can sharpen your skills in communicating and dealing with conflict.

Table 23-1
The Directions and Tactics in Conflicts

Direction 1:
Avoiding the Conflict
Tactics:

(a) Postponement.

(b) Arguments and discussions about "how to proceed in resolving the conflict."

(c) Resorting to use of formal rules.

(d) Precueing — giving prior clues about your position so the other person knows what to expect. This defuses the intensity of the issues.

(e) Keeping the track of gripes and grievances which later are "dumped" on the other person. The following discussion or arguments concern the gripes rather than the more basic differences.

(f) Coercive, strong-arm tactics—including bribes. These squelch the opposition and hence avoid issues.

(g) Refusal to recognize the conflict.

Direction 2:

Maintaining the Conflict
Tactics:

(a) Striking a bargain. Each side gives something to please the other and maintain the status quo, but the real issue of conflict is not resolved. (A couple, for example, may decide to live together "because of the kids" but their marital difficulties are not solved.)

(b) Combining escalation and reduction tactics.

Direction 3:
Escalating the Conflict
Tactics:

(a) Name-calling (describing another person or issue as "communistic," "rigid," etc.).

(b) Issue expansion (pulling in other issues to increase significance of

the conflict).

(c) Coalition formation (finding other people to serve as allies which increases your power).

(d) Threatening.

(e) Constricting the other person (frustrating a person by cutting off discussion, announcing time limitation, etc.) This increases the other person's tendency to fight back.

(f) Personal Attack.

Direction 4:
Reducing the Conflict
Tactics:

(a) Fractionation (breaking the conflict into smaller issues and dealing with these one at a time).

(b)Asking for more information about the other person's point of view and trying to understand.

(c) Talking about what is happening and what each is feeling as you

communicate in the conflict.

(d) Stating your own position clearly and concisely.

(e) Compromising – relying on a situation where everyone loses

something and everyone wins something.

(f) Resisting tendencies to criticize, attack, or use emotionally loaded

words (like "rigid," "unreasonable," "stupid," etc.).

Adapted with permission from Joyce Hocker Frost, and William W. Wilmont, Interpersonal Conflict (Dubuque, LA: William C. Brown Co. Publishers 1978)

Table 23-2
Guidelines for Communication

1.   Remember that actions speak louder than words;

nonverbal communication usually is more powerful than verbal communication. Avoid "double messages" in which the verbal and nonverbal messages convey something contradictory.

2. Define what is important and stress it; define what is unimportant and deemphasize or ignore it. Avoid fault-finding.

3. Communicate in ways that show respect for the other person's worth as a human being. Avoid statements which begin with the words "You never…"

4. Be clear and specific in your communication. Avoid vagueness.

5. Be realistic and reasonable in your statements. Avoid exaggeration and sentences which begin with the words "You always…"

6. Test all your assumptions verbally by asking if they are accurate. Avoid acting   until this is done.

7. Recognize that each event can be seen from different points of view. Avoid assuming that other people see things like you do.

8. Recognize that your family members and close friends are experts on you and your behavior. Avoid the tendency to deny their observations about you— especially if you are not sure.

9. Recognize that disagreement can be a meaningful form of communication. Avoid destructive arguments.

10. Be honest and open about your feelings and viewpoints. Bring up all significant problems even if you are afraid that doing so will disturb another person. Speak the truth in love. Avoid sullen silence.

11. Do not "put down" and/or manipulate the other person with tactics such as   ridicule, interrupting,

name-calling, changing the subject, blaming, "bugging," sarcasm, criticism, pouting, guilt-inducing, etc. Avoid the "one-upmanship" game.

12. Be more concerned about how your communication affected others than about what you intended. Avoid getting bitter if you are misunderstood.

13. Accept all feelings and try to understand why others feel and act as they do. Avoid the tendency to say "you shouldn't feel like that."

14. Be tactful, considerate, and courteous. Avoid taking advantage of the other person's feelings.

15. Ask questions and listen carefully. Avoid preaching or lecturing.

16. Do not use excuses. Avoid falling for the excuses of others.

17. Speak kindly, politely, and softly. Avoid nagging, yelling, or whining.

18. Recognize the value of humor and seriousness. Avoid destructive teasing.

Adapted with permission from Joyce Hocker Frost, and William W. Wilmont, Interpersonal Conflict (Dubuque, LA: William C. Brown Co. Publishers 1978)

PREVENTING POOR INTERPERSONAL RELATIONS

How do you prevent poor interpersonal relations? Christianity, more than any other religion, is a religion of interpersonal relationships. It all began in Genesis, when God promised a redeemer for fallen man. This was validated and manifested when Jesus, the Christ, was crucified and rose again—triumphant over death, hell, and the grave.

God is love. You and I are supposed to communicate

that love. How do we do it? By having good interpersonal relationships.

There are some guidelines in the Bible for preventing poor interpersonal relationships. There is I Corinthians 13, the "Love Chapter" for starters. Then, we must be good models ourselves and teach others to consistently follow the teachings of the Bible on how to live; pray daily; study the Bible; seek divine guidance; and conduct a self-inventory on a continuing basis in an effort to cultivate those attitudes, beliefs, confessions and actions that will please God.

This is the way to hang up the Hang-up of poor interpersonal relations.

HANG-UP NUMBER TEN:
Deliverance

No doubt this title raises many questions. "What is deliverance?" "Why is a psychiatrist writing about deliverance?" "I thought deliverance had to do with delivering people from the bondage of Satan. What is this subject doing in a book like this?"

When I thought about the subject I, too, wondered why God wanted me to include a chapter on this subject. As I continued to look to Him, He told me. I hope this comes across to you as you continue to read.

God has shown me that deliverance is a major part of the ministry of the Body of Christ. He reminded me that approximately one-fourth of His earthly ministry was involved with deliverance. Then He revealed to me how Satan had been mocking man, mocking psychiatrists in their efforts at helping those in trouble.

Here is an example of what I mean. Some of my co-workers and I were called upon to see a young woman from a nearby town who had been having emotional problems for some time. There had been no help from the psychiatrists or others she had consulted. Her marriage and family life were being destroyed. Those who tried to minister to her spiritually were baffled by the on-again, off-again attitude of the young woman.

Later I learned that she had been seeing a psychiatrist who said she had a "multiple personality." While the psychiatrist had this young woman under hypnosis, "another" personality had spoken to him. This situation aroused my interest since I had read a number of articles in psychiatric journals about this subject, complete with patient history and an account of the encounter with the "multiple personality."

As I was pondering this part of the lady's history,

the Holy Spirit spoke to me and said, "That is a demon, or an evil spirit that lives in that young woman, who is oppressing her," and by accident the doctor had bumped into him.

In our dealing with this young woman, during her actual deliverance, we, too, talked with this "multiple personality." We obtained his identity and learned that he was an evil spirit come to oppress and harass this lady. During the three hours that my co-workers and I worked with her in spiritual warfare, we cast a number of these demons out of her, in the Name of Jesus.

You may say, "Do you claim that in this day of enlightenment, in modern America, that the devil oppresses or possesses people?" Yes, that is exactly what I am saying.

You might then say, "But I thought we only heard about these things in the 'backward' nations of the world— in the jungles of Africa, South America and other places where people are primitive and worship demon spirits."

Open your eyes and look around you. How much emphasis do you see on the occult? You see it everywhere. We name cars after it. We name cereal after it. We wear occult jewelry. We read our horoscopes every day to be sure we behave right and make the right choices so we will have good fortune. Why does the primitive tribesman in South America or Africa wear occult jewelry? He, too, is taken up with the occult, with fortunetelling.

What are some of the popular television shows and movies? For example, one show that was popular a few years ago was "I Dream of Jeannie," where the main character was a young lady who was a witch—a genie. Now there is a movie called "Bewitched," where again the main character is a young wife who is a witch and whose mother also is a witch.

What kind of music do we listen to? Rock and Roll.

Did anyone ever tell you that this is a street term for illicit sexual relations? Have you bothered to listen to the lyrics of rock and roll songs? They are filthy, speaking about death, suicide, drugs, and sexual perversions.

Where do you suppose all this garbage comes from? Certainly not from God or God's people. It is from Satan. The Bible quotes Jesus as stating that "Satan came to kill, to steal and to destroy, but I come to give life and that more abundantly," (John 10:10). It is very easy to tell what God is associated with and what Satan is associated with. This scripture tells you how to distinguish God's work from Satan's.

Who do you think promotes and directs all the crime in the world? That answer should be easy: Satan. Many people who have done terrible, awful crimes say afterward, "I don't know what made me do it. Something just seemed to come over me." There are indeed two forces at work in the world today: Satan who comes to kill, steal and destroy, and Jesus, who comes to give abundant life.

God has pointed out to us in His Word all that we need to know about Satan and how to defeat him. We can study the Bible and learn how to overcome Satan every day.

The young woman's "multiple personality" and her deliverance made me want to know more about spiritual warfare and deliverance. Here are the results of my study as revealed to me from God's Word as well as from other writers who have studied this same subject.

The work of Satan can be aptly illustrated by four scriptures.

Lying Promises -- **Genesis 3:5**
"For God knows that when you eat of it your eyes will be opened, and you will be as God, knowing good and evil." Was this true? Certainly not. Did eating the forbidden fruit

make Adam and Eve like God? Certainly not. Did they know good and evil? Certainly not. Disobeying God's instructions only produced guilt and fear. Satan lied. He is the author of lies. He is speaking his native tongue when he lies. His plan is to kill, steal and destroy.

Misusing the Scriptures -- **Matthew 4:6**
"If you are the Son of God, he said, throw yourself down. For it is written: He will command his angels concerning you and they will lift you up in their hand, so that you will not strike your foot against a stone." Here Satan is quoting Psalm 91:11-12, but he is misusing the scripture. God didn't say "Go climb up on the temple steeple and cast yourself down." Yet, Satan implies that is the meaning of this scripture. He twisted it; he misused it. Jesus showed Satan up with his answer by replying, "It is also written, do not put the Lord your God to the test." Satan quoted the scripture rightly, but he misused it by distorting its meaning.

Cunning Plans -- **2 Corinthians 2:11**
"Lest Satan should get an advantage of us: for we are not ignorant of his devices." Satan is cunning, but we are aware of his schemes and are able to recognize him for what he is and what he is doing.

Appearing as an Angel of Light – **2 Corinthians 11:14**
"And no marvel; for Satan himself is transformed into an angel of light."

These four methods are Satan's wiles—his schemes

to seduce and corrupt mankind and put them into bondage. Many people are fooled by Satan and allow him to rule over them. Satan has only one weapon: deception. He uses this weapon with great skill.

When Adam sold out to Satan and did what Satan suggested (only to learn that he had been deceived), he made all mankind subject to Satan's deceptive influence. Adam gave Satan dominion over this planet. Satan is an illegal alien; he was not born on this planet like you and me. Jesus came and restored our rights on planet earth. He gave back to us the dominion that Adam sold out.

Through Jesus, we have victory over our most powerful enemy, Satan. Jesus tells us that we have His Name, His Blood, His Word and the power of the Holy Spirit. Through them we can cast out demons. In fact, deliverance is part of the great commission Jesus left to every believer. Jesus expects us to carry out this part of the great commission just as much as preaching the gospel to save sinners.

Here are some scriptures that illustrate this expectation:

Luke 10:18-19
"And he said unto them, I beheld Satan as lightning fall from heaven. Behold, I give unto you power to tread on serpents and scorpions, and over all the power of the enemy: and nothing shall by any means hurt you."

Mark 16: 17
"And these signs shall follow them that believe; In my name shall they cast out devils; they shall speak with new tongues."

Revelation 15:2

"And I saw as it were a sea of glass mingled with fire: and them that had gotten the victory over the beast, and over his image, and over his mark, and over the number of his name, stand on the sea of glass, having the harps of God."

Ephesians 4:27

"Neither give place to the devil."

Ephesians 6:10-11

"Finally, my brethren, be strong in the Lord, and in the power of his might. Put on the whole armour of God, that ye may be able to stand against the wiles of the devil."

James 4:7

"Submit yourselves therefore to God. Resist the devil and he will flee from you."

I Peter 5:8-9

"Be sober, be vigilant; because your adversary the devil, as a roaring lion, walketh about, seeking whom he may devour: Whom resist stedfast in the faith, knowing that the same afflictions are accomplished in your brethren that are in the world."

Satan has no authority over the believer because he is a defeated foe. We must take authority over him, cast him down, cast him out, and treat him as Jesus did. As **Luke 10:19** says, "Nothing shall by any means hurt you."

What are some of the indications that you are probably dealing with satanic bondage or influence? There are several of them

96

1. Emotional or Mental Problems -- Fear, phobias, depression, rebellion, anger, hatred, violent temper, jealousy, feelings of inferiority or insecurity, doubts that are difficult to shake, feelings of rejection

2. Sex Problems -- All kinds of sex problems such as homosexuality, fornication, adultery, incest, provocativeness, masturbation, lust, fantasy sexual experiences and perversions

3. Addiction Problems -- alcohol, drugs, gambling, overeating (gluttony)

4. Speech Problems -- extreme profanity, lying, criticism, mocking, railing, gossiping, and stuttering

5. Physical Diseases -- Many physical ailments are due to a Spirit of Infirmity or a Spirit of Affliction.

6. Religious Error -- any kind of involvement with religious error can open the door for demons to oppress and even possess a person. Even objects and the literature associated with religious error can attract demons. Let's name a few of these religious errors.

> (a.) False Religions – eastern religions, pagan ceremonies and philosophies, and mind sciences including physical activities such as yoga and karate. The last two practices are associated with heathen worship, of which much is satanic.

> (b.) "Christian" Cults – such as Christian Science, Rosicrucians, Unity, Jehovah's Witnesses, Mormonism. Under this also could be included some lodges and social clubs which use scripture and even God as a foundation but they omit the

atonement of Jesus for our sins with His precious blood.

(c.) The Occult and Spiritism – such as witchcraft, magic, séances, ouija boards, levitation, palmistry, handwriting analysis, E.S.P., hypnosis, automatic handwriting, astrology, horoscopes, divination and many more.

(d.) False Doctrine – **I Timothy 4:1** warns against being led astray by false teachings. We should heed this admonition.

Involvement in these practices opens the door to demon oppression and even possession.

I cannot hope to cover this subject in one chapter in this book. There are many good books available on the deliverance ministry. These texts will give more detail as well as instruction and Biblical foundation for dealing with Satan and his bondage of human beings. One book I recommend is *Demons and the World Today* by Merrell F. Unger as it goes into detail on dealing with demonism and deliverance.

The question always arises, Can a Christian have a demon? The answer is Yes. Can a Christian be possessed by Satan? I do not believe that Satan can possess the spirit of the born again Christian because possession means ownership. A Christian's mind and body can be oppressed and severely influenced by evil spirits or satanic spirits. The non-Christian has little defense against Satan's wiles. Much of the suffering, sickness, and depravity of mankind today can be attributed to demonic influence.

In her book, *Pigs in the Parlor*, Ida Mae Hammond shares what God, through the Holy Spirit, revealed to her about schizophrenia—its causes and how it works. The Holy Spirit told her that this illness was caused by demons or an inward interlocking of demon spirits. He revealed that these demon spirits usually enter a person's life when they are very young. Two major spirits involved are Rejection and Rebellion. These form the "core" of the demon spirits that indwell the schizophrenic and represent two personalities: a rejection personality and a rebellion personality. All of the evil spirits are under the control of a demon called "Schizophrenia" or "Double-mindedness."

Schizophrenia always begins with rejection. Later on, rebellion becomes evident. A schizophrenic person really has three personalities: in addition to these two, there is the real personality.

How does a schizophrenic person come out of this situation? Mrs. Hammond notes how God showed her that the three main areas which have to be conquered are Rejection, Rebellion, and the Root of Bitterness. All of these evil spirits have to be cast out of a person. With the person's cooperation and persistent determination, all the demons can be cast out and the real personality can rise up. As these spirits are conquered, the other related spirits lose their hold and strength. As this process is continued over a period of time, the individual can gain deliverance and healing.

In these days just before Christ's return, God is revealing many things to the members of the Body of Christ. God is out to defeat Satan and to perfect His Church. To do that, the Body of Christ must learn how to deal with Satan and how to defeat him in every area of man's existence. God is a good God. He wants to heal and deliver everyone.

There are many questions about deliverance that can be asked. Some of them have no complete answer. On the other hand, there are honest differences of opinion among those who are recognized authorities in this ministry.

I believe that just as the great commission commissioned you and me to preach the gospel to every creature, it also directs us to cast out devils. Just as the great commission is to every believer, so the task of deliverance belongs to every believer.

Every believer in the Body of Christ needs to be aware of Satan's wiles and deceptions and be prepared to do battle or spiritual warfare with Satan. Ephesians 6:10-18 describes our equipment and tells how we can win the battle. **Luke 10:19** says that we have authority over <u>all</u> the power of Satan and nothing shall by any means harm us.

Let me encourage you to get into the Word. Learn how to take your authority as a child of God and cast out Satan. Cast Satan out of your own life and family, and help set other captives free. Then you will be able to hang up this Hang-up.

Dr. Rufus E. Medlin

BIBLIOGRAPHY

The Twelve Rules for Raising a Delinquent. Developed by the Houston Texas Police Department. USA.

Pigs in the Parlor. Ida Mae Hammond, Impact Christian Books, Inc. USA

TO HIS GLORY PUBLISHING COMPANY, INC.

463 Dogwood Dr. Lilburn, GA. 30047, U.S.A (770)458-7947

Order Form for Bookstores in the USA

Order Date: ....

Order Placed By: ....   By fax: ....

Address: ....   By phone: ....

....

City .... ST/ZIP ....   Terms: ....

Phone#: ....

Email: ....   Discount: ....

Purchase Order#: ....

Return Policy: Within 1 Year but not before 90 days

Title and ISBN#

Price	Quantity	List Price
Shipping Method:		
Media		
UPS		
FedEx		
Other (please describe) Total Price:	Total Quantity:	

Ship To Address: Bill To Address:

TO HIS GLORY PUBLISHING COMPANY, INC. (770) 458-7947 Use Only - Billing Information

Dr. Rufus E. Medlin

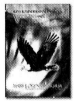
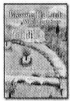
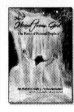
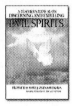

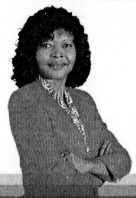
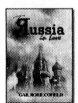

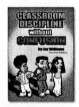

Printed in the United States
47355LVS00001B/157-312